Emily Gilmore

INTERMITTENT FASTING: THE PERFECT DIET

A Complete Easy Guide to Lose Weight, get Healthy, Strong and Slim again without Feeling Hungry.

Table of Contents

viii

Chapter 1: What is Intermittent Fasting and its Types

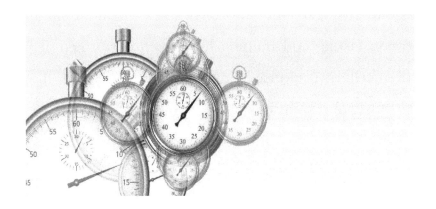

Intermittent fasting involves alternating periods of eating and prolonged fasting. A plan that has positive benefits for losing weight and living longer.

Fasting alone does not help to detoxify the body, since organs, such as the liver, which perform the task of disposing of toxins, need fuel, or rather nutrients, to function properly. Instead, carefully regulating food intake can have a positive effect.

Therefore, Intermittent fasting is the perfect solution.

Fasting causes a stress that leads cells to develop strengthening mechanisms. It can be compared to a workout that, through damage creation, leads the body to become stronger and more resilient. The similarities between fasting and training have been confirmed at the level of cellular response by numerous studies. What allows for a positive response is the possibility that the body will recover. This is why intermittent fasting seems to be the best.

When you stop fasting, no matter what Intermittent Fasting pattern you follow, the body learns to make good use of fat reserves. Together with an adjustment of the insulin response, the cells start a repair process, which brings benefits especially in the long run.

Intermittent fasting is not as hard as you may think. If anything, it is the exact opposite. There is less planning involved, and many people who have practiced it say that they feel more energetic and generally good during the fast.

It may be challenging when starting, but the body quickly adapts, and you get used to it.

Types of Intermittent Fasting

The most popular types of intermittent fasting are:

16/8 Method

The sixteen is the number of hours you're likely to be fasting, that may also be lowered to twelve or perhaps fourteen hours if that fits into your life better. Then your eating period is going to be between eight and ten hours every day. This might seem daunting, but it just means that you are skipping an entire meal. You can begin your fast around 7 or 8 p.m. and then do not eat until 11 or noon the next day: you fast for the recommended 16 hours without too stress since you are sleeping during the most of the time. The next day you can eat dinner and the day after do not eat again until lunch, skipping just breakfast. As you see, it's not so bad as it seems.

Lean-Gains Method (14:10)

Through this method, you fast anywhere from 14 to 16 hours and spend the remaining 10 or 8 hours each day engaged in eating and exercise. This method features fasting and eating during the same day, so that you don't have to be quite cautious about extending the physical effort to exercise on the days you are fasting because those days when you're fasting are every day!

20:4 Method

For the 20:4 method, you'll fast for 20 hours each day and squeeze all your meals, all your eating, and all your snacking into 4 hours. You can have two smaller meals or just one large meal and a few snacks during the 4-hour window to eat.

Meal Skipping

Meal skipping is an extremely flexible form of intermittent fasting that can provide all of the benefits of intermittent fasting but with less of the strict scheduling.

It is important to realize that you may not always be maintaining a 10-16-hour window of fasting with meal skipping. As a result, you may not get every benefit that comes from other fasting diets. However, this may be a great solution to people who want an intermittent fasting diet that feels more natural.

Warrior Diet Fasting

The most extreme form of intermittent fasting is known as the Warrior Diet. This intermittent fasting cycle follows a 20-hour fasting window with a short 4-hour eating window. During that eating window, individuals are supposed only to consume raw fruits and vegetables. They can also eat one large meal. Typically, the eating window occurs at nighttime so people can snack throughout the evening, have a large meal, and then resume fasting.

Because of the fasting length of the Warrior Diet, people should also consume a fairly hearty level of healthy fats. Doing so will give the body something to consume during the fast to produce energy with. A small amount of carbohydrates can also be incorporated to support energy levels, too.

Eat-Stop-Eat (24 Hour) Method

The eat-stop-eat method involves one to two days a week being 100% oriented towards fasting, with the other five to six days concerning "business as normal." The one or two days spent fasting are then full 24-hour days spent without eating anything at all. These days, of course, water and coffee are still fine to drink, but no food items can be consumed whatsoever. Exercise is also frowned upon on those fasting days but see what your body can handle before deciding how that should all work out.

Alternate-Day Method

The basic idea is that you fast on one day and then eat what you want the next day.

Alternate-day fasting is a solid place to start from, especially if you work a varying schedule or still have to get used to a consistent one. If you want to make things more intense from this starting point, the alternate-day method can easily become the eat-stop-eat method, the crescendo method, or the 5:2 method. Essentially, this method is a great place to begin.

12:12 Method

As another of the more natural ways of intermittent fasting, 12:12 approach is well-suited to beginning practitioners.

Many people live out 12:12 method without any forethought simply because of their sleeping and eating schedule but turning 12:12 into a conscious practice can have just as many positive effects on your life as the more drastic 20:4 method claims.

Chapter 2: Setting Goals

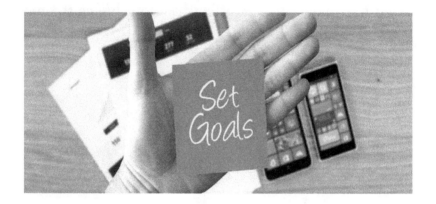

Set Goals

A healthy weight loss goal is to lose between one and two pounds every week. If you start losing more, there's a chance that you are losing muscle mass. There's credible research to confirm that it's possible to lose lean muscle mass with Intermittent Fasting if you don't eat enough protein. The goals with Intermittent Fasting depend on your health and weight goals. You can determine your diet goals by answering a couple of simple questions:

Which improvements are you seeking? Do you want to:

- Reduce the symptoms of illness,
- Feel better,
- Become more energized,
- Lose weight, or
- All of the above?
- Are you interested in practicing the diet long-term, or only until you meet your goals?
- How will you track the intake of macronutrients?
- What are your diet preferences?

Calculate Body Mass Index

Body Mass Index or BMI is an indicator of whether your current weight is healthy compared to your height. You can calculate your BMI by dividing your weight in kilograms by your squared height (m). If your results are between 18.5 and 24.9, you are healthy. Anything below 18.5 isn't healthy. The ideal measure is 21 for women and 23 for men.

However, this calculation doesn't account for body fat, waist circumference, eating habits, and lifestyle. All of this goes into how healthy you are.

Your BMI can be higher if you are masculine, which doesn't mean that you should lose weight if you are healthy. You can think of yourself as obese if your BMI is over 30. However, this isn't exclusive to the number because it's possible to have a healthy weight with an unhealthy body fat. These are rough calculations that can cause you to think of Athletic and someone who is thinner but has more body fat as obese. However, calculating your BMI can help you determine your weight loss goals in collaboration with your doctor and a dietitian.

Calculate the Body Fat Percentage

Looking into your body-fat percentage will help you to understand what you should do to lose weight, for example:

- Which method of Intermittent Fasting is the most appropriate?

- Whether or not you want to incorporate the Keto diet in the Intermittent Fasting?

- How much do you need to exercise, and what kind of exercises are necessary?

If you like exercising, Intermittent Fasting will help you lose body fat, but preserve or gain muscle mass. As a result, you may not notice scaling down. However, even if you don't lose weight, but gain muscle mass, you will still look slimmer.

To track how your body fat changes, you can use the body composition scales. These scales help you track how your muscle mass, your hydration, and your body fat change throughout your diet.

Calculate Waist-To-Hip Ratio

The waist-hip ratio or WHR is a more credible measurement because it accounts for your natural body shape. For women, an ideal measure is 0.8, while 0.9 is ideal for men. If your measurements are higher, you should work on your shape.

For calculating the WHR, you can use a tape measure and measure the circumference of the widest part of your hips and your natural waist, which is slightly above your belly button. After that, divide your waist measurement by your hip measurement.

Plan Your Portions

Calculate Basal Metabolic Rate

While measuring meals isn't required with Intermittent Fasting, it is desirable to maintain optimal health levels. To start, you should calculate your basal metabolic rate to find out how many calories you need to maintain your weight, and how many you need to lose it.

Calculate the Right Portion Sizes

When calculating portion sizes, keep in mind that 1 gram of nutrients translates to a different number of calories:

- Fat-9 calories,

- Protein- 4 calories, and

- Carbohydrate-4 calories.

Calculate the Daily Calorie Intake

In general, Intermittent Fasting doesn't require calorie restriction for weight loss. Still, weight loss and other health benefits of fasting will be greater if you have a controlled daily calorie intake.

Chapter 3: Rules to Follow to Lose Weight

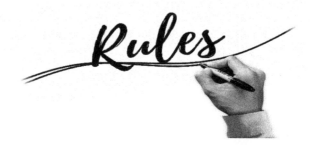

It is very important to reiterate that proper transition into an intermittent fasting lifestyle is very important.

It is a Lifestyle Change

A very important thing that people easily and most often overlook is that intermittent fasting is just not staying hungry for a few hours a day. It is a complete lifestyle change. As you are reading this book, you might find it very easy. It can't be too difficult to stay hungry for 12-16 hours. Believe me; it isn't. However, when you need to respect that limitation for months and years, it can look difficult. Most people don't go that far. They start finding it difficult within a week or a month at the most.

Eliminating snacks from your routine will be the hardest decision you'll make. Not having anything voluntarily and not being able to have anything are two very different things.

Most people fail in their weight loss journey because first, they believe that things are very easy and then come under the impression that they are very difficult. The truth lies somewhere in-between.

1. You must start with the elimination of snacks.

2. Follow this routine for so long that you don't feel the need to have snacks

3. Then, begin placing three nutrient-dense meals within an eating window of 12 hours

4. Follow this routine until you're are well adjusted to it.

5. Increase your fasting hours to 14.

6. Follow this routine for at least a quarter

7. Begin shifting your breakfast as closer to lunch as possible without putting too much strain on your body

8. At this stage, you must not set a goal for fasting hours. Just don't eat as long as you don't feel really hungry

9. You must also keep in mind not to starve yourself when feeling hungry

10. Only stick to a longer fast if you are comfortable with it and never rush with any step on the way

It Only Looks Easy

This is very important learning you must keep with yourself. Intermittent fasting only looks easy, but it is a lifestyle that needs to be practiced. Even with intermittent fasting, you will experience frustrating moments when you wouldn't want to move ahead. You must never take it for granted.

Following a routine with discipline is difficult, and training yourself to follow it with precision is always a challenge. If you want to succeed in your goals, you must plan.

Plan your steps

Step One — Create a Monthly Calendar

On a calendar, highlight the days you wish to fast, depending on the type of fast you have committed yourself to. Record a start and end time on your fasting days, so you know how you plan to begin and finish in the days leading up to your fast day.

19

Tick off your days; this will keep you motivated and on track!

Step Two — Record Your Findings

Create a journal for your fasting journey. One or two days before the time, undertake to do your measurements. Weigh yourself first thing in the morning, after you have gone to the restroom and before breakfast. Also, do not weigh yourself wearing heavy items as they may affect the outcome of the scale.

Measure your height as this figure is related to your BMI (body mass index) result.

Record the measurements around your hips and stomach area, if you wish, you can also measure your upper thighs and arms.

Take a photo of yourself and place it into the journal too; this is not to discourage you but to keep you focused on why you began this journey.

20

Jot down all of these findings and update them weekly in the journal.

A journal is also the perfect way to express how you are feeling and, of course, what you are most thankful for. A journal is an important way to track not just the physical aspects of the diet but also its mental aspects. Never undertake to doubt yourself; your journal should be a safe space for you to congratulate and to motivate yourself. Leave all the negative thoughts at the door!

Step Three — Plan Your Meals

The easiest way to stick to any eating program is to plan your meals; 500 calorie meals tend to be simple and easy to create but there are also many other more complex recipes for those who wish to spice things up. Who knows, perhaps you stumble across a meal you wish to eat outside of your fasting days.

It is advised that you prepare your meals the day before your fast days; doing this helps you stay committed to the fast and limits food wastage.

Initially, and in the first few weeks, it is suggested that you keep your meal preparation and recipes simple, so as not to overcomplicate the whole process. This also allows you to get used to counting your calories and knowing which foods work to keep you fuller versus those that left you feeling hungrier earlier than later.

Be sure to include your meal plan in your journal and on your calendar.

Step Four — Reward Yourself

On the days where you may return to normal eating, it is important to reward yourself. A small reward goes a long way in reminding yourself and your brain that what you are doing has merit and that it should be noticed.

A reward should cater to one of our primal needs; these needs include:

- Self-actualization
- Safety needs
- Social needs
- Esteem needs

Physiological needs such as food, water, air, clothing, and shelter.

Have a block of chocolate or buy yourself a new item of clothing to do anything that makes your heart happy!

Step Five — Curb Hunger Pains

Initially, you will feel more discomfort when hungry, but these feelings will pass. If you do find yourself craving something, sip on black tea or coffee to help you through your day. Coffee is known to alleviate the feelings of being hungry; if you must add sweetener, do so at your discretion.

Know that some sweeteners can cause the opposite effect and make you feel hungry.

Step Six — Stay busy

Keeping busy means that the mind does not have time to dwell on your current state of affairs, especially if you find yourself reaching for a snack bar or cookie.

It is also wise to be implementing some sort of physical activity, even on your fasting days. A 20-minute walk before ending your fasting period will do wonders to help you reach the final stages of the fasting period. It can also uplift your mood when you are feeling frustrated or tense.

Step Seven — Practice Mindful Eating

As mentioned, we are inclined to eat for all sorts of reasons; happy, sad, it does not matter. The problem is that these feelings related to food become habitual, so we aren't really hungry, but we seek to tuck into something delicious because we feel good or even off.

The art of eating mindfully is not to allow these habits to master your life. The concept is simple: teach yourself to look at something, for instance, a piece of cake and think, "Do I need it or do I want it for other reasons?" You could decide to have a bite or two and leave the rest, but you may be less inclined to eat the whole slice (or whole cake) if you think mindfully about it.

The art of mindful eating is to revel in the food placed before you. Pay attention to colors, textures, and tastes. Savor each bite, even when eating an apple.

Your brain gradually begins to rewire itself when it comes to food and when it needs or wants something.

Practice mindful eating by:

- Pay attention to where your food comes from.
- Listen to what your body is telling you; stop eating when you are full.

- Only eat when your body signals you to do so; when your stomach growls or if you feel faint or if your energy levels are low.

- Pay attention to what is both healthy and unhealthy for us.

- Consider the environmental impact our food choices make.

- Every time you take a bite of your meal, set your cutlery down.

Step Eight — Practice Portion Control

Controlling portion sizes can be difficult for most; society has also regulated us to what we think is the size of an average portion. We have access to supersizing meals too, which does not help those struggling in the weight department. In 1961, Americans consumed 2,880 calories per day; by 2017, they consumed 3,600 calories, which is a 34% increase and an unhealthy one at that.

To help you navigate how to portion your food better, consider trying the following: when dishing up your food, try the following trick. Half of your plate should consist of healthy fruits and/or vegetables, one quarter should be made up of your starches such as potatoes, rice, or pasta, and the remaining quarter should be made up of lean meats or seafood.

Alternatively, try the following:

- Dish up onto a smaller plate or into a smaller bowl.
- Say no to upsizing a meal if offered.
- Buy the smaller version of the product if available or divide the servings equally into packets.
- Eat half a meal at the restaurant and take the remaining half to enjoy the following day instead.
- Go to bed early; it will stop any after-dinner eating.

Step Nine - Get Tech Savvy

Modern-day society has plenty to offer us in terms of the apps we can use to help determine the steps we take, the calories we burn, the calories found in our foods, research, information, and motivation for lifestyle changes, especially diets and exercise. The list is endless. There are many apps on the market currently that can help you track your progress about fasting.

The best intermittent fasting apps of currently (at the time of writing), and in no particular order are:

- Zero
- Fast Habit
- Body Fast
- Fasting
- Vora
- Ate Food Diary

Life Fasting Tracker

Make use of your mobile device to set reminders for yourself when to eat, what to eat, and when your fast days are. It works especially well when using it to set reminders when you should drink water, particularly for those who find it hard to keep their fluids up.

Making the Change

Understand that intermittent fasting is not a diet; it is a lifestyle, an eating plan that you are in control of, and one that is easy to perfect. Before you know it, fasting will become second nature.

When to Start?

Begin today, not tomorrow or after a particular event or gathering. Once you have picked the fast that best suits you, begin with it immediately. Never hold off until a specific day; once you begin, you will gain momentum and it will become something that is part of your day, like many other things that fill up your day. No sweat there!

Measure Your Eating

Three days before you fast, it would be wise to begin to lessen the amount of food you are eating or dishing up less. This helps your body begin to get used to the idea that it doesn't need a whole bowl of food to get what it needs or feel full.

Keep up Your Exercise Plan

If you have a pre-existing exercise regime, do not alter it anyway. Simply carry on the way you were before fasting. If you are new to exercising, begin with short walks now and again, extending the time you walk. For example, take a five-minute walk, and the next day, change the time to 10 minutes of walking.

Stop, Start, Stop

Fast for hours, and then eat all your calories during a certain number of hours. Consider this as a training period.

Do Your Research

Read up as much as you can about intermittent fasting this way, it will put to rest any uncertainties you might have and introduce you to new ways of getting through a fasting day.

Check out recipes that won't make you feel like a rabbit having to chew on carrots all day if you are stuck with ideas of what to eat.

Have Fun

Lastly, have fun, and see what your body can do, even over 50. It is important to know that just because you are a certain age doesn't mean you are incapable of pursuing a new lifestyle change. Reward yourself when it is due, track your progress, adjust where the need is, and get your beauty sleep. This is another secret to achieving overall wellness and happiness.

Know Your BMI

Your BMI is based on your weight and height; thus, you can easily determine your body mass index, or BMI as it is more commonly known.

In total, there are four categories that an individual can fall into based on this figure. That is underweight, healthy, overweight, and obese. The concept is simple: our BMI gives us quantifiable amounts when comparing our height with our fat, muscles, bones, and organs.

How to Calculate Your BMI

To calculate your BMI, equate your weight (lbs.) x 703 divided by your height (in).

Once you have calculated your BMI, you can compare it to the body mass index chart to determine which category you are classed into.

Class	Your BMI Score
Underweight	less than 18.5 points
Normal weight	18.5 – 24.9 points
Overweight	25 – 29.9 points
Class 1 — Obesity	30 – 34.9 points
Class 2 — Obesity	35 – 39.9 points
Class 3 — Extreme obesity	40 + points

Chapter 4: What to Eat and Not to Eat During Intermittent Fasting

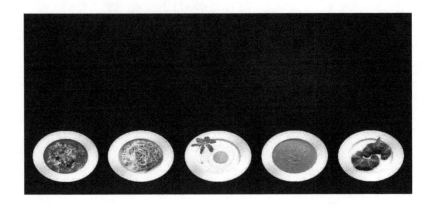

No matter how you plot your path when it comes to an intermittent fast, you need to have an understanding of what is good to eat, and not to eat during your efforts. Unless you are engaging in a complete fast from solid foods for 24 hours, you will have to know just what you should eat on your fast days. Likewise, it would be good to know what might be best suited for your non-fast days too. Because remember, just because you might be on one of your non-fast days, doesn't mean it would be a good idea to go downtown and binge at all you can eat buffet. Here in this chapter, we will help guide you to make wise food choices on what to eat and what not to eat during your intermittent fasting.

What to Eat

Coffee

Coffee as a zero-calorie beverage is a great supplement to any fast day since it can help to ameliorate possible negative reactions to fasting. If your initial fast has you feeling a bit lethargic and lacking in energy for example, a good stiff cup of coffee could certainly help to offset those symptoms.

Raspberries

Raspberries are a low-calorie food that won't wreck your fast day and at the same time, will help keep you regular by giving you healthy dose of fiber. Raspberries also come replete with healthy vitamins and minerals, as well as inflammation busting antioxidants. In some situations, raspberries are even said to prevent cancer. This is due to a powerful cancer busting phytochemical it boasts, called "ellagic acid."

36

Low Calorie Beans and Legumes

Beans, beans, the magical fruit. The more you eat, the more fat you can burn for your fast. Both beans and legumes are packed with healthy nutrients and are typically low in calories. They also have plenty of protein, helping to keep your muscles fueled even while your fat stores are depleted. Tiny but mighty, beans and legumes are fully capable of aiding in the process of weight reduction, during your intermittent fast. Most especially good when it comes to intermittent fasting are peas, black beans, lentils, and garbanzo beans.

Blueberries

These fruitful treats are low in calories yet high in antioxidants, helping to ensure the body remains free of nasty free radicals that could degrade bodily tissue over time. Blueberries are known immune boosters too, good for ensuring you don't get sick or otherwise compromised while you fast. Another neat thing about blueberries is that they contain a little something called flavonoids, which if consumed over a long period of time, can work to reduce overall BMI (Body Mass Index).

Eggs

Egg is a great low calorie, nutrient dense food for your fast days. Eggs have a ton of proteins and tend to stick with you, leaving you filling full and satisfied.

Lean Chicken Breast

If you aren't doing a 24 hour fast, a serving of lean chicken breast is a good way to end a fast day that shouldn't exceed your 500-calorie allotment. Lean chicken breast provides plenty of proteins without all the filler of other sides of meat.

Fish

Just like chicken, fish is a good source of protein and yet won't break your budget of allotted calories on your fast day. Fish has a ton of what are known as omega-3 fatty acids. Don't let the "fat" word scare you thought, because omega-3 fatty acids are a good thing: they can safeguard our heart, dramatically reduce blood pressure, clear out plaque from arteries, and even prevent heart attacks and strokes. Fish is also considered a "brain food" due to its ability to help enhance cognitive function.

Veggies

As well as providing plenty of valuable nutrients, veggies also give us a healthy dose of fiber to help keep us regular. Vegetables are typically low in calories too, so you can mix and match them with all kinds of meals regardless of meal plans.

Whole Grains

Whole grains are a great source of nutrition on fast or non-fast day either one. Unlike refined grains that spike your insulin, these morsels won't make you mess up your fast, and will still leave you feeling full and satisfied.

Yogurt

Yogurt is an excellent source of nutrients and also provide a boost to your metabolism and energy even as you fast. Yogurts also come complete with a dose of probiotics that once ingested will work around the clock to keep your gut in good shape. The experts are stressing more and more that so-called good gut bacteria is the key to good health.

Dark Chocolate

Dark chocolate gives you a boost of energy even while fortifying your system with valuable antioxidants. The kind of antioxidants capable of fighting off cancer no less.

Coconut Oil

Coconut oil is a low calorie, known metabolism booster, and will get your system up and running during your period of intermittent fasting. Coconut oil is good because it doesn't trigger insulin production unlike other oils do. You can use coconut oil as a supplement, or even a cooking aid, without any fear of disrupting your fast in the process.

What Not to Eat

Soda

One of the major components of an intermittent fast after all, is the avoidance of sugar. It's so your body will start burning fat stores already in place that during fasting we refrain from guzzling sugary soda for our metabolic rate to nibble on.

Heavily Processed Food

Anything that has been processed and packaged is going to have a ton of preservatives packed into them, that while generally harmless, will have a long-term effect on your system over time. Heavily processed food will also pose a direct interference with your metabolism.

Sugary Sweets

Just like with sugary sodas, sugary sweets would be completely counterproductive for an intermittent fast. The goal of an intermittent fast after all is to switch the body from burning sugar and carbs, to burning our latent fat deposits instead. Eating sugary sweets would disrupt this process and instead just add more junk to the fat already deposited in our trunk.

Alcohol

Alcohol and intermittent fasting do not mix. The reason? Alcohol has a direct effect on fat burning metabolism. And the last thing that you would want to do is wreck your fast by throwing a wrench in your fat burning metabolism! Alcohol also carries, carbs, sugars, calories and the like.

Refined Grains

Refined grains once metabolized will actually turn directly into sugar. As already mentioned, the whole purpose of intermittent fasting is to get your body to stop burning sugar as fuel and burn fat instead. Ingesting refined grains that turn into sugar therefore, completely negates this process. It will also raise your insulin levels.

Trans-Fat

Trans-fat, the fatty acids found in certain milk and meat products should be avoided. It raises, cholesterol, insulin, and wrecks any chance you may have had of having a successful fast.

Fast Food

Even though we call it "fast food"—the burgers and fries we bag from places like McDonald's are not exactly the best thing to eat during an intermittent fast! One look at an overly processed, carb dense meal from McDonald's and I think you might probably understand why.

Chapter 5: Intermittent Fasting & Keto Diet: The Perfect Duo

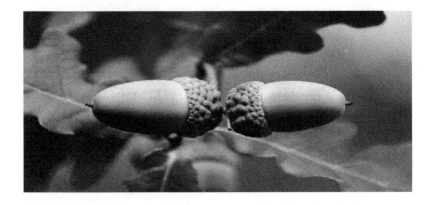

The ketogenic diet offers many of the same benefits associated with intermittent fasting, and when done together, most people will experience significant health improvements, including not just weight loss. The ketogenic diet and intermittent fasting allow the body to move from a state where sugar is burned to a state where fat is burned (important flexibility, which in turn promotes optimal cell function and body systems). And although

46

there is evidence that the two strategies work independently, I understand that the combination of the two strategies provides the best results overall.

There are at least two important reasons to favor the pulse approach. Insulin deactivates liver gluconeogenesis, that is, the production of glucose by the liver. When insulin is chronically suppressed for long periods, the liver begins to compensate for its lack by producing more glucose. As a result, your blood sugar starts rising even if you don't eat carbohydrates.

More importantly, in general many metabolic benefits associated with nutritional ketosis actually occur during the re-feeding phase. In the fasting phase, the removal of damaged cells and their contents occurs, but the real rejuvenation process takes place during refeeding. In other words, the cells and tissues are rebuilt, and their healthy state is restored when the intake of net carbohydrates increases. (Rejuvenation during re-feeding is also one of the reasons why intermittent fasting has so many benefits, because you cycle hunger and abundance.)

How to Apply Cyclic Ketosis And Fasting?

1. Take an intermittent fasting program - eat all meals (from breakfast to lunch, or from lunch to dinner) within an eight-hour time frame each day. Fast for the remaining 16 hours. If all of this is new to you and the idea of making changes in your diet and eating habits scares you too much, simply start by eating your usual meals during this time. Once it becomes a routine, continue implementing the ketogenic diet, and then making it cyclical. You can find comfort in knowing that once you reach the third step you can replenish some of your favorite healthy carbohydrates on a weekly basis.

If you want to maximize the health benefits of fasting further, consider switching to regular five-day fasting on water alone. For example, I do it three or four times a year. To simplify this process, gradually reach a point where you fast for twenty hours a day and eat two meals in just four hours. After a month, fasting while consuming only water for five days will not be that difficult.

2. Switch to a ketogenic diet until you generate measurable ketones - the three main stages are: limit the net carbohydrates (total carbohydrates without fiber) from 20 to 50 grams per day; replace the eliminated carbohydrates with healthy fats in in order to obtain 50 to 85% of the daily caloric intake from fats and limit the protein to half a gram for every half kilo of lean body mass.

Avoid all trans fats and polyunsaturated vegetable oils that are not fine. Adding these harmful fats can cause more damage than excess carbohydrates, so just because a food is "high in fat" doesn't mean you should eat it. Keep these portions of net carbohydrates, fats and proteins until you get into ketosis and your body burns fat as an energy source. To determine that you are ketotic, you can use the ketone test strips, checking that the ketones in your blood are in the range of 0.5 to 3.0 mmol / L.

Remember that precision is important when it comes to portions of these nutrients. In fact, an excess of net carbohydrates will prevent ketosis as the body will first use any available glucose source, being a type of fuel that burns faster. Since it is practically impossible to determine the amount of fat accurately, net carbohydrates and proteins in all dishes, make sure you have some basic measuring and tracking tools at your fingertips.

3. Once you have verified you are in ketosis, start cycling in and out of ketosis by replenishing high amounts of net carbohydrates once or twice a week. As a general recommendation, the amount of net carbohydrates triples during the days you fill up on carbohydrates.

Remember that the body will again be able to effectively burn fat at any time after a couple of weeks or a few months. As already mentioned, entering and exiting cyclically from nutritional ketosis will maximize biological benefits of regeneration and renewal, while at the same time minimizing potential negative sides of continuous ketosis. At this point, even if high or low carbohydrates are given once or twice a week, I would still advise you to be careful about what is healthy and what is not.

Chapter 6: Tips and Tricks to Start And Follow The IF

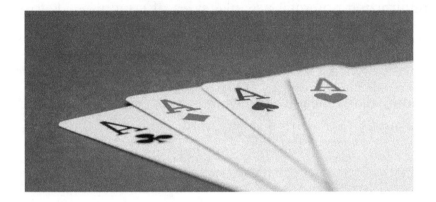

Intermittent fasting is not easy. We need support as much as possible and anything that can make your journey easier. Below are some of the tips that will make your journey smooth and effective.

Decide on your fasting window.

Intermittent fasting is not a strict time-based diet. This means that you can choose the number of hours to fast and when to fast either day or night. The fasting and eating window periods are not a must to be the same every day.

Ensure you get enough sleep.

When you get enough sleep, you become healthier, and your overall well-being is guaranteed. When we sleep, the body operates certain functions in the body that helps burn calories and improves the metabolic rate.

Eat healthy Avoid eating anything you want after a fast.

Healthy meals should be your focus. They will help you get the required nutrients like vitamins, which will give you more energy during the fasting period.

Drink more water.

One of the best decisions you can make during a fast is to drink water. It will keep your body hydrated and taking water before meals can significantly reduce appetite.

Start small.

If you have never tried it before, there is no way you start fasting and go for a whole 48 hours without a meal. For beginners, you can start by having your food at 8 pm, for example, and having nothing again until 8 am the next day. It will be easier since sleep is incorporated in your eating window.

Avoid stress.

Intermittent might be hard to do if you are stressed. This is because stress can trigger an overindulgence of food to some people. It is also easier to feed on junk when stressed to feel better. That's why when on intermittent fasting, you are advised to avoid if not control your stress levels.

Be disciplined.

Remember that fasting means the abstinence of food until a particular time. When fasting, be true to yourself and avoid eating before the stipulated time. It will ensure that you lose maximum weight and benefit health-wise from intermittent fasting.

Keep off flavored drinks.

Most flavored drink says that they are low in sugar, but in the real sense, they are not. Flavored drinks contain artificial sweeteners, which will affect your health negatively. They will also increase your appetite, causing you to overeat, and this will make you gain weight instead of losing.

Find something to do when fasting.

It is said that an idle mind is the devil's workshop. When you are on intermittent fasting and not busy, you will be thinking about food, and this will make you break your fast before the stipulated time. You can keep yourself busy by running errands, listening to music, or even taking a walk in the park.

Exercising

Exercise can be done when fasting, but it is not a must. Mild exercises can be done even at home. By exercising, you will build your muscle strength, and your body fat will burn faster.

Chapter 7: Most Common Mistakes and How To Avoid Them

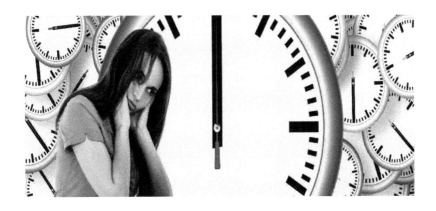

When you are looking to make any significant adjustments in your life, it can take time to discover exactly how to do it in the best ways possible. Many people will make mistakes and have some setbacks as they seek to improve their health through intermittent fasting. Some of these mistakes are minor and can easily be overcome, whereas others may be dangerous and could cause serious repercussions if they are not caught in time.

In this chapter, we are going to explore common mistakes that people tend to make when they are on the intermittent fasting diet. We will also explore why these mistakes are made, and how they can be avoided. It is important that you read through this chapter before you actually commit to the diet itself. That way, you can ensure that you are avoiding any potential mistakes beforehand. This will help you in avoiding unwanted problems and achieving your results with greater success and fewer setbacks.

You should also keep this chapter handy as you embark on your intermittent fasting diet. That way, if you do begin to notice that things are not going as you had hoped, you can easily reflect back on this chapter and get the information that you need to adjust your diet and improve your results.

Switching Too Fast

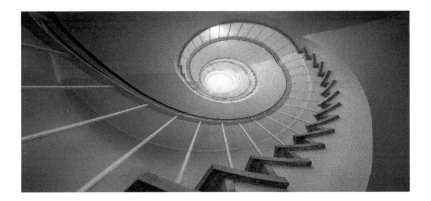

A significant number of people fail to comply with their new diets because they attempt to go too hard too fast. Trying to jump too quickly can result in you feeling too extreme of a departure from your normal. As a result, both psychologically and physically you are put under a significant amount of stress from your new diet. This can lead to you feeling like the diet is not actually effective and like you are suffering more than you are actually benefitting from it.

If you are someone who eats regularly and who snacks frequently, switching to the intermittent fasting diet will take time and patience. I cannot stress the importance of your transition period enough.

It is not uncommon to want to jump off the deep end when you are making a lifestyle change. Often, we want to experience great results right away and we are excited about the switch. However, after a few days, it can feel stressful. Because you didn't give your mind and body enough time to adapt to the changes, you ditch your new diet in favor of things that are more comfortable.

Fasting is something that should always be acclimated to over a period of time. There is no set period, it needs to be done based on what feels right for you and your body. If you are not properly listening to your body and it needs you are going to end up suffering in major ways. Especially with diets like intermittent fasting, letting yourself adapt to the changes and listening to your body's needs can ensure that you are not neglecting your body in favor of strictly following someone else's guide on what to do.

Choosing the Wrong Plan for Your Lifestyle

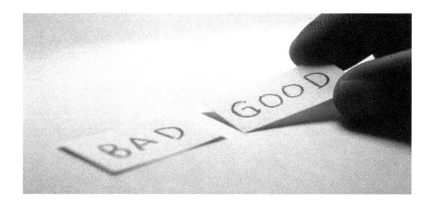

It is not uncommon to forget the importance of picking a fasting cycle that actually fits with your lifestyle and then fitting it in. Trying to fast to a cycle that does not fit with your lifestyle will ultimately result in you feeling inconvenienced by your diet and struggling to maintain it.

Often, the way we naturally eat is in accordance with what we feel fits into our lifestyle in the best way possible. So, if you look at your present diet and notice that there are a lot of convenience meals and they happen all throughout the day, you can conclude two things: you are busy, and you eat when you can. Picking a diet that allows you to eat when you can is important in helping you stick to it. It is also important that you begin searching for healthier convenience options so that you can get the most out of your diet.

Anytime you make a lifestyle change, such as with your diet, you need to consider what your lifestyle actually is. In an ideal world, you may be able to adapt everything to suit your dreamy needs completely. However, in the real world, there are likely many aspects of your lifestyle that are not practical to adjust. Picking a diet that suits your lifestyle rather than picking a lifestyle that suits your diet makes far more sense.

Taking the time to actually document what your present eating habits are like before you embark on your intermittent fasting diet is a great way to begin. Focus on what you are already eating and how often and consider diets that will serve your lifestyle. You should also consider your activity levels and how much food you truly need at certain times of the day. For example, if you have a spin class every morning, fasting until noon might not be a good idea as you could end up hungry and exhausted after your class. Choosing the dieting pattern that fits your lifestyle will help you actually maintain your diet so you can continue receiving the great results from it.

Eating Too Much or Not Enough

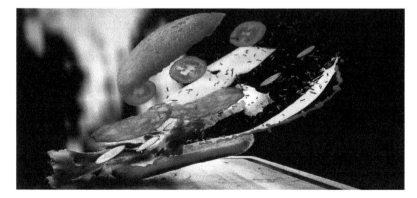

Focusing on what you are eating and how much you are eating is important. This is one of the biggest reasons why a gradual and intentional transition can be helpful. If you are used to eating throughout the entire day, attempting to eat the same amount in a shorter window can be challenging. You may find yourself feeling stuffed and far too full to actually sustain that amount of eating on a day to day basis. As a result, you may find yourself not eating enough.

If you are new to intermittent fasting and you take the leap too quickly, it is not unusual to find yourself scarfing down as much food as you possibly can the moment your eating window opens back up. As a result, you find yourself feeling sick, too full, and uncomfortable. Your body also struggles to process and digest that much food after having been fasting for any given period of time. This can be even harder on your body if you have been using a more intense fast and then you stuff yourself. If you find yourself doing this, it may be a sign that you have transitioned too quickly and that you need to slow down and back off.

You might also find yourself not eating enough. Attempting to eat the same amount that you typically eat in 12-16 hours in just 8-12 hours can be challenging. It may not sound so drastic on paper, but if you are not hungry you may simply not feel like eating. As a result, you may feel compelled to skip meals. This can lead to you not getting enough calories and nutrition in on a daily basis. In the end, you find yourself not eating enough and feeling unsatisfied during your fasting windows.

The best way to combat this is to begin practicing making calorie-dense foods before you actually start intermittent fasting. Learning what recipes you can make and how much each meal needs to have in order to help you reach your goals is a great way to get yourself ready and show yourself what it truly takes to succeed. Then, begin gradually shortening your eating window and giving yourself the time to work up to eating enough during those eating windows without overeating. In the end, you will find yourself feeling amazing and not feeling unsatisfied or overeating as you maintain your diet.

Your Food Choices are Not Healthy Enough

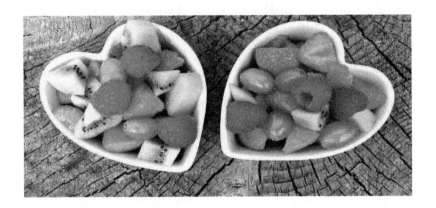

Even if you are eating according to the keto diet or any other dietary style while you are intermittently fasting, it is not uncommon to find yourself eating the wrong food choices. Simply knowing what to eat and what to avoid is not enough.

You need to spend some time getting to understand what specific vitamins, and minerals you need to thrive. That way, you can eat a diet that is rich in these specific nutrients.

Then, you can trust that your body has everything that it needs to thrive on your diet.

Even though intermittent fasting does not technically outline what you should and should not eat, it is not a one-size-fits-all diet that can help you lose weight while eating anything you want. In other words, excessive amounts of junk foods will still have a negative impact on you, even if you're eating during the right windows.

It is important that you choose a diet that is going to help you maintain everything you need to function optimally. Ideally, you should combine intermittent fasting with another diet such as the keto diet, the Mediterranean diet, or any other diet that supports you in eating healthfully. Following the guidelines of these healthier diets ensures that you are incorporating the proper nutrients into your diet so that you can stay healthy.

Eating the right nutrients is essential as it will support your body in healthy hormonal balances and bodily functions. This is how you can keep your organs functioning effectively so that everything works the way it should. As a result, you end up feeling healthier and experiencing greater benefits from your diet. It is imperative that you focus on this if you want to have success with your intermittent fasting diet.

You are Not Drinking Enough Fluids

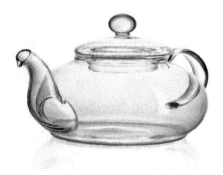

Many people do not realize how much hydration their foods actually give them on a day to day basis. Food like fruit and vegetables are filled with hydration that supports your body in healthily functions. If you are not eating as many, then you can guarantee that you are not getting as much hydration as you actually need to be. This means that you need to focus on increasing your hydration levels.

When you are dehydrated you can experience many unwanted symptoms that can make intermittent fasting a challenge. Increased headaches, muscle cramping, and increased hunger are all side effects of dehydration. A great way to combat dehydration is to make sure that you keep water nearby and sip it often. At least once every fifteen minutes to half an hour you should have a good drink of water. This will ensure that you are getting plenty of fresh water into your system.

Other ways that you can maintain your hydration levels include drinking low-calorie sports drinks, bone broth, tea, and coffee. Essentially, drinking low-calorie drinks throughout the course of the entire day can be extremely helpful in supporting your health. Make sure that you do not exceed your fasting calorie maximum, however, or you will stop gaining the benefits of fasting. As well, water should always be your first choice above any other drinks to maintain your hydration. However, including some of the others from time to time can support you and keep things interesting so that you can stay hydrated but not bored.

If you begin to experience any symptoms of dehydration, make sure that you immediately begin increasing the amount of water that you are drinking. Dehydration can lead to far more serious side effects beyond headaches and muscle cramps if you are not careful. If you find that you are prone to not drinking enough water on a daily basis, consider setting a reminder on your phone that keeps you drinking plenty throughout the day.

The best way to tell that you are staying hydrated enough is to pay attention to how frequently you are peeing. If you are staying in a healthy range of hydration, you should be peeing at least once every single hour. If you aren't, this means that you need to be drinking more water, even if you aren't experiencing any side effects of dehydration.

Typically, if you have already begun experiencing side effects then you have waited too long. You want to maintain healthy hydration without waiting for symptoms like headaches and muscle aches to inform you that it is time to start drinking more. This ensures that your body stays happy and healthy and that you are not causing unnecessary suffering or stress to your body throughout the day.

You Are Giving Up Too Quickly

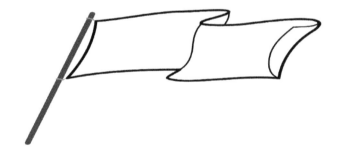

A lot of people assume that eating the intermittent fasting diet means that they will see the benefits of their eating habits immediately. This is not the case. While intermittent fasting does typically offer great results fairly quickly, it does take some time for these results to begin appearing. The exact amount of time depends on many factors. How long it has taken you to transition, what and how you are eating during eating windows, and how much activity you are getting throughout the day all contribute to your results.

You might feel compelled to quickly give up if you do not begin noticing your desired results right away, but trust that this is not going to help you. Some people require several weeks before they really begin seeing the benefits of their dieting. This does not mean that it is not working, it simply means that it has taken them some time to find the right balance so that they can gain their desired results and stay healthy.

If you are feeling like throwing in the towel, first take a few minutes to consider what you are doing and how it may be negatively impacting your results. A great way to do this is to try using your food diary once again. For a few days, track how you are eating in accordance with the intermittent fasting diet and what it is doing for you. Get a clear idea of how much you are eating, what you are eating, and when you are eating it. Also, track the amount of physical activity that you are doing on a daily basis.

Through tracking your food intake and exercise levels, you might find that you are not experiencing the results you desire because you are eating too much or not enough in comparison to the amount of energy you are spending each day. Then, you can easily work towards adjusting your diet to find a balance that supports you in getting everything you need and also seeing the results that you desire.

In most cases, intermittent fasting diets are not working because they are not being used right for the individual person. Although the general requirements are somewhat the same, each of us has unique needs based on our lifestyles and our unique makeup. If you are willing to invest time in finding the right balance for yourself then you can guarantee that you can overcome this and experience great results from your fasting.

You are Getting Too Intense or Pushing It

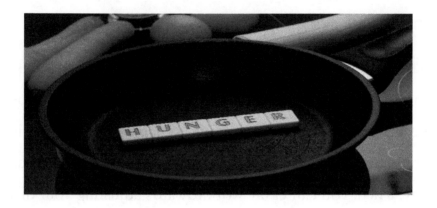

If you are really focused on achieving your desired results, you might feel compelled to push your diet further than what is reasonable for you. For example, attempting to take on too intense of a fasting cycle or trying to do more than your body can reasonably handle. It is not uncommon for people to try and push themselves beyond reasonable measure to achieve their desired results. Unfortunately, this rarely results in them achieving what they actually set out to achieve. It can also have severe consequences.

At the end of the day, listening to your body and paying attention to exactly what it needs is important. You need to be taking care of yourself through proper nutrition and proper exercise levels. You also need to balance these two in a way that serves your body, rather than in a way that leads to you feeling sick and unwell. If you push your body too far, the negative consequences can be severe and long-lasting. In some cases, they may even be life-threatening.

In some cases, pushing your body to a certain extent is necessary. For example, if you are seeking to build more muscle then you want to push yourself to work out enough that your workouts are actually effective. However, if you are pushing yourself to the point that you are beginning to experience negative side effects from your diet, you need to draw back. While certain amounts of side effects are fairly normal early on, experiencing intense side effects, having side effects that don't go away or having them return is not good. You want to work towards maintaining and minimizing your side effects, not constantly living alongside them. After all, what is the point of adjusting your diet and lifestyle to serve your health if you are not actually feeling healthy while you do it?

Make sure that you check in with yourself on a daily basis to see to it that your physical needs are being met. That way, if anything begins to feel excessive or any symptoms begin to increase, you can focus on minimizing or eliminating them right away. Paying close attention to your needs and looking at your goals long-term rather than trying to reach them immediately is the best way to ensure that you reach your health goals without actually compromising your health while attempting to do so. In the end, you will feel much better about doing it this way.

Chapter 8: Intermittent Fasting and Working Out

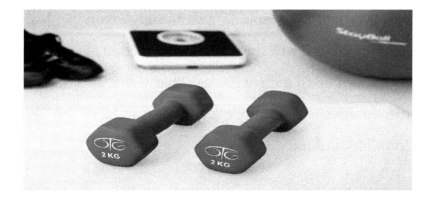

If food is your source of fuel, should you be exercising without it?

There are some people who keep their workout routine quite basic, taking the idea of being active as taking a walk or cleaning their house. Then there are people who follow their gym workout routines planned out five to six days a week and never skip a workout. They get their cardio in daily and combine it with weights. Some even tend to think of themselves as full-on bodybuilders.

When you reach the point that all you want to do is be the fittest you can be and thrive off it, it is a wonderful thing. Suddenly, losing weight or maintaining your goal weight and physique isn't such a difficult thing to do, and you hardly ever feel like skipping a workout. Anyone with that type of mentality will find that losing weight is extremely easy and not at all a difficult task that waits for you either before or after work in the evening. It's, in fact, something to look forward to.

However, for the average individual, working out may not be so fun and easy to do. It may seem like something you dread thinking about from the early hours of the morning to the evening when you finally reach your hour of working out.

Now, for those who don't take their workouts too seriously, not eating before a workout, like in the morning once you wake up, will seem relatively easy. That is, if you're going to walk your dog or consider vacuuming your carpet as a workout. On the other hand, if you feel like you need your fuel for a workout, should you be planning your meals around it to suit your needs or try something different?

Exercising on an Empty Stomach

Since your body makes use of stored carbohydrates, otherwise known as glycogen, when working out to provide you with energy, you should know that there's no need to eat before working out. In fact, at some point, you may have heard that fasted workouts are much better for fat loss than working out after eating. Working out during a fasting period can help you burn up to 20% more fat than if you ate breakfast before a morning workout.

That's because, after fasting for eight to 12 hours, your body taps into its fat stores. So, when you're working out during your fasting period, you are burning fat instead of calories because your calories have already been depleted. This promotes a leaner body and provides you with all the energy you need to get through your workout.

If you feel like you're really struggling to work out on an empty stomach, consider cutting your fasting period, perhaps from 16 hours to 10 or 12 hours. You can also take BCAA's to provide you with a proper boost of energy for your workout. Finally, you can try drinking a cup of coffee 15 to 30 minutes before working out.

Anyone that feels they just can't work out on an empty stomach or feel weak when doing so should opt for a workout in the afternoon or before their last meal of the day.

Is There a Safe Way to Exercise While Intermittent Fasting?

If you're interested in working out while integrating intermittent fasting into your daily schedule, there are a few things to consider first.

Research has proven that exercising after eating before the digestion of food takes place is necessary for anyone suffering from metabolic syndrome or type 2 diabetes. In that same breath, research also suggests that exercising when fasting every day can affect the biochemistry of your muscles, along with your metabolism (Weatherspoon, 2018).

Since your glycogen stores are likely to be depleted after fasting, you are, once again, more able to burn fat as fuel instead of calories. While it is believed that we can burn more fat on an empty stomach, there is more to learn before you dive into your fasted workouts.

Intermittent fasting combined with exercising for an extended period isn't considered a good thing, according to Priya Khorana, PhD, the Columbian University nutrition educator. Studies also suggest that there is a big chance of your metabolism slowing down as a result of long-term fasting. However, it can help you burn more fat for a certain period at a time (Weatherspoon, 2018).

During fasting, you can burn more fat, but unless it is suited for you, you may not perform as well as you normally would during your workouts. During your fasting period, unless your diet accommodates your workout routine, you could lose muscle mass. You could potentially also be able to maintain your current muscle mass, yet not be able to build more muscle.

To ensure you're working out safely while fasting, you should keep a schedule of your day. With intermittent fasting, it's very important to make your workout as effective as possible during fasting. Consider when it is the right time to exercise. This, of course, will depend on the type of fasting method you're following. If you only have an 8-hour window to fuel up on food, you may want to work out before you break your fast. Anyone focused on performance and recover should work out on an empty stomach on the 16:8 fasting method to achieve lean muscle mass and burn fat.

When working out, it doesn't matter what type of diet you're following, you must choose the diet that suits the macronutrients you take before you work out. Consider only doing strength workouts on the day after you consume a lot of carbs. With cardio or short bursts of high-intensive training, like HIIT, however, you can do this on a low-carb day.

The best way to look after your body during intermittent fasting, to build lean muscle and avoid injuries, is to eat a healthy, balanced, and fueling meal after your workout. After an intense strength training workout, it is necessary to fuel up on up to 20 grams of protein and an adequate amount of carbs in a 30-minute window after your workout.

Other than that, be sure to stay hydrated and drink plenty of water during the day, eat a high-protein meal directly after your workout, push your electrolytes, and above all else, listen to your body.

Chapter 9: Simple to Follow Exercises

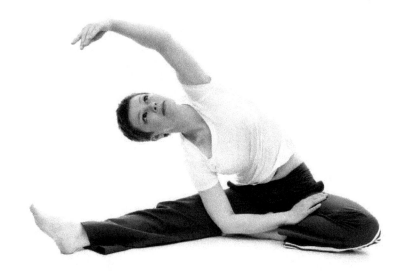

Yet many may wonder if it's safe to exercise during an intermittent fast. With the body depleted of nutrients during a fast after all, would it be wise to put it through any more strain than it's already under? According to the data, exercise while undergoing a fast has a direct effect on metabolism and the body's level of insulin. Both are activated with one going up and the other going down as the body recalibrates and begins to burn fat rather than carbs. Engaging in the right kind of workout will help to speed up this process even more. Having that said, here are some exercises to give your intermittent fast a major boost.

Running/Treadmill

There is really nothing better to get the body's metabolic cylinders running than a good run. As soon as your feet hit the pavement (or the treadmill), your heart rate increases, and the blood starts to much more vigorously pump through your body. With your bodily processes instantly speeding up like this, it's really no wonder that your metabolism might speed up as well. And this is precisely the case when you engage in this type of exercise during a fast. But having that said, just keep in mind that you have to be careful not to overdo it. And in order to ensure that you have the best experience, it is recommended that you only run during the first few hours of your fast. That way your body still has plenty of additional resources left over from the last meal you had before your fast began. If for example you began your fast at 10 PM on a Thursday night, you should be good to run around the block at 7AM Friday morning without any trouble. It is not advisable however to overexert yourself at the very end of your fast. Although most could probably handle it, just to be on the safe side, you should keep your running hours locked into the first few hours of your fast. Every step you take causes hormones to alert your metabolic engines that you are up and quite literally running.

Weightlifting

If you are a weightlifter, or interested in becoming one—I have some good news for you. Lifting weights does not interfere with your fast! In fact, lifting weights during a fast can prove quite beneficial. As mentioned previously in this book, the very style of intermittent fasting is designed to prevent muscle loss during fasting periods, but having that said, a little weightlifting will help to shield your body from muscle loss even more. Because the truth is, we all lose muscle as we age and if we don't work at maintaining it through muscle lifting, we just might find that our muscle mass declining significantly through the years. Even more beneficial for those wishing to lose weight, lifting weights during an intermittent fast also quickens the pace of fat burn even more. Just think about it, during a fast your body has already switched to burning fat for its fuel, so when you grunt, struggle, and strain to lift those weights, guess what your body's tapping into for energy? All that fat you want to get rid of! Do I dare say—this is a win win situation? It most certainly is!

Pushups

One of the most traditional exercises you could ever even consider would be that of the classic pushup. Pushups have been around forever and there is a reason for that—they are highly effective. By making use of gravity and your own body weight, the push up gets the heart going while the muscles do overtime to push the body up off the floor by virtue of arm strength alone. These exercises if done moderately—say no more than 20 to 30 pushups during a fast—can be highly effective in boosting your metabolism to the max, allowing an even more rapid depletion of the body's fat stores. This is some good news that you could most certainly use!

Squats

This is another great exercise that seems absolutely made for intermittent fasting. Squats focus on your glutes, quads and other muscles like there is no tomorrow! This exercise keeps you going and keeps you strong! As you might imagine, squats consist of the participant bending their knees and squatting down toward the ground as if they are sitting on a chair. This bending motion gets the blood flowing to the thighs and begins rapidly burning fat deposits. If you need to target fat in the legs in particular, you might want to give this exercise a try.

Dips

Why yes—we would be remiss if we did not mention dips! And no, I'm not talking about the stuff you dip your chips in at the football game, I'm talking about high intensity, fat busing exercise that will burn fat, boost your metabolism and make sure your upper body stays nice and strong. These exercises are just about perfect for intermittent fasting as they get the blood flowing without making you too tired in the process.

Planks

Planks are a fairly common yet highly efficient exercise that can be done at home, at the gym, or just about any place you may be at the time. This exercise is also quite nuanced and flexible when it comes to adjusting the intensity and the area of focus. Planks tend to build up quite a bit of endurance too, which is most certainly good for someone who is undergoing a fast. It is best to engage in this exercise during the first few hours of your fast, but they can be done periodically throughout the rest of the fasting day as well.

Reverse Lunge

This exercise may look easy at first glance but don't be fooled. Reverse lunges are a high intensity workout that gets your metabolism going. And when done during a fast, it really kicks things into high gear. They are also good for getting your legs in tip top shape which is beneficial for just about every other aerobic exercise you could do.

Burpee

No, a burpee isn't what happens when you eat too many hot peppers. A bad joke maybe, but in all seriousness, there are many out there who are confused with what a burpee is and what it is not. The Burpee is a classic hybrid styled exercise that makes full use of cardio as well as resistance exercises, in order to maximize your metabolism. These exercises are pretty intensive, so if you are engaged in a less than 500 calorie fast day, you might want actually to have a low-calorie snack or other healthy option. Good choices for nutrition before this workout would be perhaps just a 1 hard-boiled egg, a salad, or maybe even a bowl of chicken broth. Either way, these workouts are sure to get your body running on all cylinders during your intermittent fast.

CPSIA information can be obtained
at www.ICGtesting.com
Printed in the USA
BVHW051554090321
602118BV00004B/373